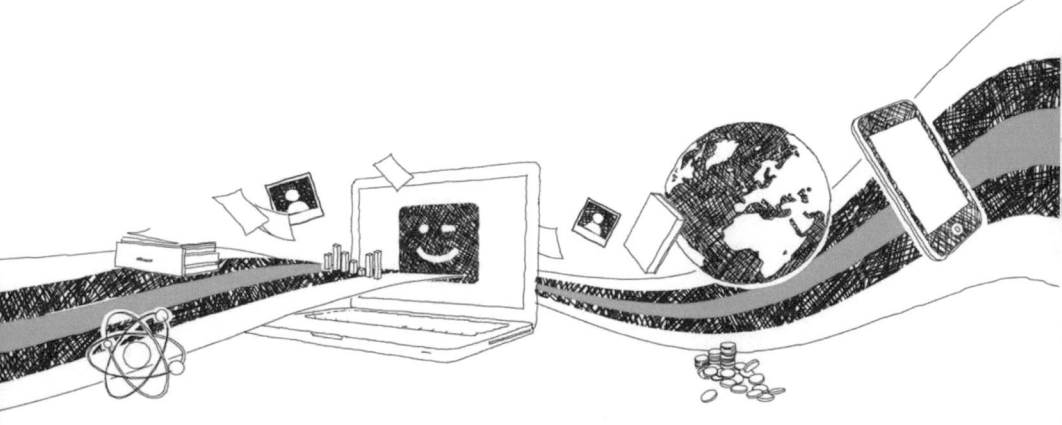
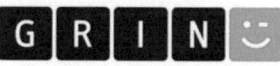

Maureen Muthoni

Bio-psychological Analysis of Autism

GRIN Publishing

Bibliographic information published by the German National Library:

The German National Library lists this publication in the National Bibliography; detailed bibliographic data are available on the Internet at http://dnb.dnb.de .

Imprint:

Copyright © 2015 GRIN Verlag GmbH
Print and binding: Books on Demand GmbH, Norderstedt Germany
ISBN: 978-3-656-93501-8

This book at GRIN:

http://www.grin.com/en/e-book/295291/bio-psychological-analysis-of-autism

GRIN - Your knowledge has value

Since its foundation in 1998, GRIN has specialized in publishing academic texts by students, college teachers and other academics as e-book and printed book. The website www.grin.com is an ideal platform for presenting term papers, final papers, scientific essays, dissertations and specialist books.

Visit us on the internet:

http://www.grin.com/

http://www.facebook.com/grincom

http://www.twitter.com/grin_com

Bio-psychological Analysis of Autism

Autism is a neuropsychological disorder that is characterized by impaired communication, social interaction, as well as restricted and repetitive behavior. Most parents usually note signs of autism in the first two years of their children's life (Le Breton, 2010). These signs usually develop gradually, but some children suffering from autism usually reach the usual developmental milestones at a relatively normal pace then start regressing. Autism is characterized by particular set of behaviors and is also a spectrum disorder. This means that autism affects individuals differently and with varying degrees and intensity. As such, while all people with this disorder share some difficulties, their condition affects them in different ways. Some behaviors associated with autism include difficulty in holding a conversation or making eye contact, delayed learning of language, difficulty with executive functioning that relates to planning and reasoning, narrow and intense interests, poor sensory sensitivities, as well as poor motor skills (Dawson, 2011). Again, an individual on the spectrum of this disorder might follow most of these behaviors or just a few of them, or many others besides. This paper critically analyses autism including its causes, pathology, treatment options, as well as the diagnostic and technologies that are employed in clinical diagnosis, care, and basic science research of this order.

History of Autism

Long before autism was named, a few examples of autistic symptoms, signs and treatments had already been described. For instance, Martin Luther's Table Talk tell a story of a twelve year old boy who was showing signs of severe autism. However. The earliest case of autism that is well-documented is that of Blair Hugh of Borgue, which is put together in a 1747 court case. Blair's brother petitioned to annul his marriage so as to gain Blair's inheritance. His petition is said to have been successful. Another historical example of autism is shown by a feral child who was caught in 1798 showing significant signs of the disorder (Dawson, 2011). However, the feral child was lucky since he was treated by Jean Itard who was a medical student. Itard treated him using a behavioral program that was designed to help the feral child form social attachments, as well as induce speech through imitations.

It was not until the year 1938 that the word autism took its modern sense. This happened when Hans Asperger, a lecturer at the Vienna University Hospital, used the terminology during a lecture about child psychology in German. At the time, Asperger was trying to investigate a particular Autism Spectrum Disorder, which is today known as sperger syndrome. In English, the term autism was first used in its modern sense by Leo Kanner who was responsible for introducing early infantile autism in the year 1943. Kanner's report highlighted eleven children who had behavioral similarities. Most of those characteristics described in that report are still considered typical for autism spectrum disorders.

In the beginning of the late 1960s, this disorder was established separately from other syndromes by demonstrating that autism is lifelong. These characteristics typical of autism distinguished it from schizophrenia, intellectual disability, and other developmental disorders. It is around the same time that clinicians and therapists started demonstrating the benefits of involving both the parents and their autistic children in active programs of therapy. As the mid and late 1970s fast approached, evidence of genetic role in pathology of autism was still scattered. Currently, autism is considered as one of the most heritable among all psychiatric conditions. My decision to tackle this particular disorder is influenced by the fact that my two year son is autistic. Therefore, I have personal experience in handling children who have autism. Again, I feel that I need more enlightenment on this disorder so that I can gain knowledge on how best to help and handle my son, as well as support him.

Last year, the Center for Diseases Control and Prevention issued a report suggesting that the prevalence of autism had increased to 1 in 68 births in the U.S alone, and 1 in 54 boys in the country. Worldwide, the rate of autism prevalence is approximated to be about one to two in every one thousand people. In addition, autism occurs 4-5 times more in boys than it does in girls (Center for Diseases and Control (CDC) , 2014). Diagnosis of autism is based on behavior of an individual, not on the mechanism or the cause since it is a spectrum disorder and its symptoms affect individuals differently. In the DSM-IV-TR, autism is defined as exhibiting about six symptoms that include at least two in impairment of social interaction, difficulties in communication, as well as another one in restricted and repetitive behavior (Dawson, 2011).

Signs and Symptoms of Autism

This disorder is highly variable that first appears during childhood or infancy. Generally, autism follows a steady course lacking remission. Overt symptoms of autism gradually begin their manifestation after the six months of age. Later, these symptoms become established by the time the child turns two or three years, tending to continue through the person's adulthood, although in a more muted form. Autism is not distinguished by just by a single symptom. Instead, it is characterized by a triad of symptoms including impairments in communication, social interaction, as well as repetitive behavior and restricted interests (Akshoonoff & Pierce , 2012). Other aspects of autism such as atypical eating habits might be common among autistic individuals but they are not essential symptoms for diagnosis. Individual symptoms for autism occur mostly in the general population and seem not to associate greatly, but of course without a distinct line separating the common traits from those that are pathologically severe.

Social Development

Individuals with this disorder often show social impairments and usually lack the intuition regarding others, which many people free of autism take for granted. Such unusual social developments start becoming apparent early on in childhood. Children with autism often show diminished attention to social stimuli (Ayres , 2013). In addition, such children smile and look at other people less often. In the same breath, autistic children respond less to their name. Autistic toddlers have less turn taking and eye contact, and they lack the ability to use the simplest of movements to express themselves, pointing at things, for example. Autistic children are less likely to show social understanding, ape and respond to emotions, approach other people spontaneously, take turns with others, and communicate non-verbally (Clifford & Gevers , 2012). However, these children form strong attachment bonds with their care givers. Contrary to popular belief that most autistic children prefer to be alone, researchers opine that these children suffer from frequent and more intense loneliness than their non-autistic peers.

Communication

Most autistic individuals fail to develop enough natural speech that is required to meet their communication needs (Clifford & Gevers , 2012). Difficulties in communication may be evident from the first year of life in autistic children. Such difficulties include unusual gestures, delayed onset of babbling, unsynchronized vocal patterns, and diminished responsiveness to the world around them. As they grow up, these children are less likely to share experiences, have less diverse and frequent babbling, master word and word combinations, as well as consonants. Such children are also less likely to repeat others words, and they have their gestures less integrated with words. Autistic children often encounter difficulties in developing symbols into language and in imaginative play (Dawson, 2011).

Repetitive Behavior

Individuals with autism often display several forms of restricted or repetitive behavior. Clinicians use the Repetitive Behavior Scale-Revised (RBS-R) to examine these behaviors. They have categorized them as stereotypy, compulsive, sameness, restricted, ritualistic, and self-injury behaviors (Vandenberg , 2013). Stereotypy refers to repetitive movements such as head rolling, hand rolling, or body rocking. On the other hand, sameness displays resistance to change while self-injury includes those movements that can injure the person, such as skin-picking and eye-poking.

Epidemiology

Most recent reviews of autism estimate a prevalence of about one to two in every one thousand people. In the United States, the Center for Diseases and Control (2014) released a report showing that about twelve in every thousand children have ASD. In the United Kingdom, the NHS approximated that autism in adults stood at 1.1% for people aged eighteen years and above (Center for Diseases and Control (CDC) , 2014). The rapid increase in the number of autism cases reported is attributed to the rampant changes in the referral patterns, diagnostic practices, public awareness, as well as availability of treatment and management services (Vandenberg , 2013). Research shows that boys are at a higher risk of acquiring autism than girls. Although evidence does not suggest exactly why it is so in boys, a number of risk factors can be identified (Dawson, 2011). Great risk of autism is associated with diabetes, advanced age of parents, substance abuse, and use of psychiatric drugs, and bleeding of the mother during bleeding (Akshoonoff & Pierce , 2012). However, to mention that ethnicity, race, and socioeconomic background are not among the risk factors for autism is important.

Theories of Etiology

This disorder is highly heritable. However, the causes of autism include both the genetic susceptibility and environmental factors. In some rare cases, this disorder is associated with some of the agents that are known to cause birth defects. Other proposes environmental causes of autism are crowded by controversies. For instance, the hypotheses attributing autism to vaccines are not only biologically unlikely, but they have also been disapproved in several scientific studies (Elder, 2012). For a long time now, it has been presumed that there exists a common cause of autism at the cognitive, genetic and neural levels that often co-occur. This is because autism is regarded as a genetic basis. However, it remains unclear whether it can be explained more by rare multi-gene interactions that are of common genetics variants or by rare mutations with major mutations (Le Breton, 2010).

Autism is also suggested to be caused by synaptic dysfunction. Evidence suggests that some rare mutations lead to this disorder by disrupting specific synaptic pathways, such as the ones involved with cell adhesion. Additionally, exposure to air pollution of heavy metals and particulates during pregnancy also increases the risk of developing autism. Autism is also attributed to lifestyle. Other researchers suggest that certain factors such as particular foods, illicit drugs, and prenatal stress can lead to autism (Akshoonoff & Pierce , 2012).

No single gene in isolation has been linked to autism. However. It has often been theorized that the responsible gene for autism might be an X-linked gene because of the high ratio of males who are autistic compared to very few females (Clifford & Gevers , 2012). In fact, just a single child out of five autistic children is female. Today, most researchers opine that autism begins with a combination of environmental triggers and genetic vulnerabilities in an individual. They also hold that autism is prenatal in nature, believing that there are genetic mutations that cause autism.

Diagnosis

Diagnosis of autism is based on behavior of an individual, not on the mechanism or the cause since it is a spectrum disorder and its symptoms affect individuals differently. In the DSM-IV-TR, autism is defined as exhibiting about six symptoms that include at least two in impairment of social interaction, impairment in communication, as well as another one in restricted and repetitive behavior (Dawson, 2011). There are several diagnostic and research technologies that are used in clinical diagnosis, care, and the basic science of autism, the Autism Diagnostic Interview (ADI-R) and the Autism Diagnostic Observation Schedule (ADOS), for example. The latter is a semi-structured interview with the parent while the former uses interaction and observation with the child. The Children Autism Rating Scale (CARS) is also used in clinical environments in assessing severity of the disorder based on observation of the child. Diagnosis of autism is usually conducted by a pediatrician who starts by performing a preliminary investigation by physically examining the child and taking their developmental history.

Treatment Options

The main goals of pediatricians when treating autism in children are mainly to lessen the associated deficits and family distress, as well as increasing quality of life and improving the child's functional independence. However, there is no one autism treatment that is regarded as universally best (Ayres , 2013). Instead, treatment for autism is usually tailored to meet the needs of specific children. Sustained and intensified special education programs, as well as behavior therapy early in the children's' life can aid them in acquiring social, self-care, and job skills later on in their lives (Le Breton, 2010). Additionally, these approaches and methods help children in improving their functioning and decreasing maladaptive behaviors and symptoms severity. Such methods include applied behavior analysis (ABA), structured teaching, developmental models, social skills therapy, language and speech therapy, and occupational therapy. In addition, there are many medications used in treatment of autism symptoms including anticonvulsants or psychoactive drugs. The most common drug classes that are also used to treat ASD symptoms include stimulants, antidepressants, as well as antipsychotics (Dawson, 2011).

In conclusion, it is evident that autism can be a lifelong developmental disorder that starts being evident in very young children. Therefore, parents should be very keen in observing their children's behavioral pattern when they are very young so as to detect any symptoms that may lead to diagnosis of autism (Akshoonoff & Pierce , 2012). Such symptoms may include impairments in communication, difficulties in social interaction, and as repetitive behavior and restricted interests. As much as there is no single known cure for autism, early diagnosis and intervention measures can help autistic individuals lead a near to normal life.

References

Akshoonoff , N., & Pierce , K. (2012). Sensory processing and classroom emotional, behavioral and educational outcomes in children with autism spectrum disorder. *American Journal of Occupational Therapy*, 72:564-573.

Ayres , J. (2013). Efficacy of sensory and motor interventions for children with autism. *Journal of Autism and Developmental Disorders*, 17(1): 56-66 .

Center for Diseases and Control (CDC) . (2014). Prevalence of Autism . *Center for Diseases and Control (CDC*.

Clifford, P., & Gevers , C. (2012). A theory of mind-based social cognition training program for school aged children with pervasive developmental disorders. *Journal of Autism and Developmental Disorders*, 30(4):567-571.

Dawson, G. (2011). *Autism: Nature, Diagnosis, and Treatment.* New York, NY: Guilford Press.

Elder, J. (2012). *Different Like Me: My Book of Autism Heroes.* London: Jessica Kingsley Publishers.

Le Breton, M. (2010). *Diet Intervention and Autism: Implementing the Gluten Free and Casein Free Diet for Autistic Children and Adults : a Practical Guide for Parents.* London: Jessica Kingsley Publishers.

Vandenberg , N. L. (2013). The use of weighted vests to increase on-task behavior in children with attention difficulties. *American Journal of Occupational Therapy*, 65(6):621-628.